TABLE OF CONTENTS

Conclusion

- Leadership Reflection Tools
- Competency Frameworks
- Leadership Development Checklist

INTRODUCTION

Leading in Healthcare: Management and Leadership in the UK and Ireland

Healthcare in the United Kingdom and Ireland is undergoing profound and accelerating transformation. Systems that were once defined by stability and predictability now operate within environments marked by increased demand, constrained resources, workforce shortages, rising public expectations, global health shocks, and rapid technological advancement. Leaders at every level must navigate unprecedented complexity, while remaining steadfast in their commitment to patient safety, equity, quality, and organisational resilience.

This book has been written to support current and aspiring healthcare leaders clinical, managerial, operational, strategic, and multidisciplinary who must lead within systems that are changing faster than ever before. The intent is practical as much as conceptual: to equip leaders with the skills, tools, and perspectives they require to lead through uncertainty, build strong teams, improve services, and drive meaningful change across the UK and Irish health sectors.

Unlike traditional leadership texts, this book recognises that healthcare leadership is not abstract. It is lived in the corridors of hospitals, in community clinics, across integrated care systems, and within social care networks. It is shaped by cultural diversity, population needs, regulatory pressures, and the lived experiences of staff and service users. It requires self-awareness, emotional intelligence, political capability, cultural humility, strategic insight, and above all a deep commitment to better outcomes for patients and communities.

Why Healthcare Leadership Matters Now More Than Ever

Across both jurisdictions, several themes dominate contemporary healthcare:

- **Rising demand:** Ageing populations, chronic illnesses, mental health pressures, and widening health inequalities reshape service needs.
- **Workforce pressures:** Recruitment, retention, burnout, and staff well-being have become priority concerns.
- **Digital acceleration:** Electronic health records, AI-driven diagnostics, virtual care, and data-enabled decision-making are redefining the delivery of care.
- **System reform:** NHS England's Integrated Care Systems (ICSs), Northern Ireland's transformation agenda, Scotland's public health commitments, Wales' prudent healthcare model and Ireland's Sláintecare

reforms all emphasise integration, prevention, collaboration, and system-wide leadership.

• **Patient expectations:** Service users now expect personalised, transparent, safe, high-quality healthcare experiences.
• **Financial pressures:** Leaders must deliver more value with fewer resources, requiring sharper strategic thinking and innovation.

Meeting these challenges demands more than competent management it demands courageous, compassionate, evidence-informed leadership grounded in values, vision, accountability, and behavioural skill.

About This Book

The chapters that follow explore both the foundations and the frontiers of modern healthcare leadership. They blend practical tools with conceptual understanding, offering readers:

• Clear explanations of core management and leadership principles
• Practical examples drawn from the UK & Ireland
• Evidence-based frameworks used across NHS and HSE systems
• Case studies highlighting real organisational challenges

• Tools, checklists, models and reflection prompts leaders can apply immediately

• Guidance on leading teams, managing change, improving quality, and strengthening culture
• Insight into digital transformation, innovation, inclusive leadership, and system-wide collaboration

Each chapter is deliberately designed to bridge the gap between theory and practice. Leadership only becomes meaningful when it is applied in real contexts on wards, in boardrooms, in community settings, within networks, and across multi-agency partnerships.

Who This Book Is For

This book is written for:

• Emerging leaders stepping into supervisory or managerial roles
• Established managers seeking to deepen their impact
• Senior clinical leaders transitioning into strategic positions
• Multidisciplinary team leaders across acute, primary, community, voluntary and social care sectors
• Students and professionals undertaking healthcare management, public health, or leadership training
• Anyone seeking clarity and confidence in navigating the UK or Irish healthcare systems

A Forward-Looking Lens

Throughout the text, attention is given to the future of healthcare leadership.

Topics such as AI adoption, integrated care, trauma-informed leadership, service-user voice, workforce culture, high-reliability systems, and cross-sector partnerships are integrated not as theoretical considerations, but as operational realities shaping the next decade.

Effective healthcare leadership is no longer defined solely by technical skill or positional authority. It is defined by behaviours, relationships, self-awareness, and the capacity to influence change across complex systems. It is the ability to lead both compassionately and decisively, balancing human needs with organisational demands. It is the willingness to question, adapt, collaborate, innovate, and advocate for safer, fairer, more effective care.

This book aims to support leaders in doing exactly that.

CHAPTER 1

Understanding the Healthcare Landscape in the UK and Ireland

Healthcare in the United Kingdom and Ireland is shaped by a combination of historical legacy, political priorities, demographic change, economic pressures, and rapidly evolving models of care. For leaders working within these systems, understanding the wider landscape is not optional it is essential.

Leadership decisions are made within the context of policy, regulation, organisational culture, service-user expectations, and workforce realities. Without a strong grounding in the landscape, leaders risk making decisions that are reactive, narrow, or disconnected from strategic context.

This chapter provides a clear, practical overview of how the systems evolved, who influences them, and the major challenges and opportunities facing healthcare today. It sets the foundation for the leadership and management tools explored throughout the rest of the book.

1.1 Evolution of Healthcare Systems in the UK and Ireland

Both healthcare systems share broad principles universal access, equity, safety, and public accountability but their histories, structures, and reform pathways differ.

1.1.1 The United Kingdom

The National Health Service (NHS), established in 1948, remains one of the world's most recognised publicly funded health systems. Its three founding principles continue to shape its identity:

- Healthcare should meet the needs of everyone
- Healthcare should be free at the point of delivery
- Healthcare should be based on clinical need, not ability to pay

Over the decades, the NHS has moved through waves of reform:

Early expansion (1950s–1980s)

- Rapid growth in hospital-based medicine

- Professional autonomy as the dominant organising principle

- Limited data, performance management, or transparency

Managerial and market reforms (1990s–2010s)

- Introduction of internal markets

- Creation of NHS Trusts

- Development of commissioning structures

- Increased emphasis on accountability, targets, waiting times, and quality assurance

- Expansion of clinical governance and national standards

Integration and population health (2019–present)

- Shift from competitive models to *collaboration across systems*

- Establishment of Integrated Care Systems (ICSs) in England

- Greater emphasis on prevention, community care, digital health, and service redesign

- Workforce shortages, rising demand, and financial constraints intensifying pressure on services

Although the four nations England, Scotland, Wales, Northern Ireland share the same NHS heritage, they now operate distinct systems with different priorities, governance models, and reform trajectories.

1.1.2 Ireland

Ireland's healthcare system has undergone significant modernisation, but its evolution has differed from the UK. Historically:

- Hospital care dominated service provision

- Primary care was fragmented and under-resourced

- Access depended more heavily on ability to pay

- Regional variation in service availability was common

Major developments include:

Establishment of the HSE (2005)

The Health Service Executive centralised governance, replacing multiple regional boards.

This began Ireland's move toward greater standardisation, improved accountability, and national oversight.

Sláintecare (2017–present)

This landmark cross-party reform plan aims to:

• Shift care into the community
• Reduce waiting lists and inequity
• Expand universal access
• Strengthen prevention and population health
• Integrate health and social care
• Reduce dependence on private healthcare

Sláintecare represents Ireland's most significant reform in decades and continues to reshape leadership expectations across the sector.

Modern pressures

Ireland faces:

- Workforce shortages

- Growing demands on emergency care

- Primary care and GP recruitment challenges

- Increasing complex health needs

- Legislative strengthening of HIQA and patient safety initiatives

1.2 Key Stakeholders and Regulatory Bodies

Healthcare leaders operate in highly regulated environments with multiple influential stakeholders. Understanding these structures is crucial for effective leadership, partnership, compliance, and change management.

1.2.1 United Kingdom

Government and policy bodies

- Department of Health and Social Care (DHSC) sets national policy
- Devolved Governments – separate health strategies for Scotland, Wales, Northern Ireland
- NHS England oversees planning, commissioning, workforce, and performance

System-level structures

- Integrated Care Systems (ICSs) – coordinate health and social care across regions
- ICBs/ICPs – strategic planning, resource allocation, population health responsibility
- Trusts and Health Boards – deliver acute, mental health, and community care services

Regulators and quality bodies

- Care Quality Commission (CQC)
- NHS Improvement (now NHS England)

• National Institute for Health and Care Excellence (NICE)
• Professional regulators: GMC, NMC, HCPC, etc.

Other key stakeholders

• Local authorities
• Voluntary and community sectors
• Trade unions
• Service-user advocacy groups
• Academic and research institutions

1.2.2 Ireland

Government and policy bodies

• Department of Health – overall policy and governance
• HSE – national service delivery, operational management, workforce and performance

Regulatory and quality bodies

• Health Information and Quality Authority (HIQA) - standards, inspections, social care, HIQA licensing
• Mental Health Commission – oversight of mental health services
• Health Products Regulatory Authority (HPRA)

Professional regulators

• Medical Council
• Nursing and Midwifery Board of Ireland (NMBI)
• CORU (allied health professionals)

Other stakeholders

- Voluntary hospitals and agencies
- Primary Care Networks
- Sláintecare Programme Implementation Office
- Patient advocates and NGOs
- Trade unions (INMO, IMO, SIPTU)

Healthcare leadership requires navigating these relationships, understanding accountability lines, and building trust across multiple organisational boundaries.

1.3 Challenges and Opportunities in Today's Healthcare Systems

Both systems face significant pressures that shape leadership priorities. These challenges should not only be understood but actively inform management strategy.

1.3.1 Key Challenges

Rising service demand

- Ageing populations

- Multi-morbidity

- Mental health pressures

- Social determinants of health

- Increased public expectations

Workforce crisis

- Difficulties recruiting nurses, GPs, social care staff

- Burnout and stress across all professions

- High vacancy levels in urban and rural areas

- Increasing industrial action
  Leaders must balance service continuity with workforce well-being and retention.

Financial constraints

Both systems face:

- Escalating costs

- Infrastructure pressures

- Increased demand for community care

- Tight budgets requiring efficiency, prioritisation and innovation

Fragmentation and complexity

Despite reform efforts, silos persist across:

- Acute and primary care

- Health and social care

- Statutory and voluntary sectors

Effective leadership requires system-thinking, partnership, and integration.

Quality and safety concerns

High-profile service failures reinforce the need for:

- Strong governance

- Cultural transformation

- Learning systems

- Transparent reporting

1.3.2 Key Opportunities

Digital transformation

- Electronic health records

- Virtual care

- AI decision-support

- Remote monitoring

- Data-driven planning

Leaders must embrace digital as a core strategic enabler.

Integrated care

Closer collaboration across sectors offers:

- Better patient journeys

- Reduced duplication

- Improved population outcomes

- More sustainable care models

Prevention and population health

Sláintecare and ICS frameworks emphasise prevention, early intervention, and addressing health inequalities.

New leadership expectations

Modern leaders are expected to demonstrate:

- Compassionate leadership

- Systems thinking

- Inclusive practices

- Trauma-informed approaches

- Staff empowerment

- High emotional intelligence

Innovation culture

The constraints facing healthcare systems often drive creativity, new models of care, and community-based solutions.

Conclusion

Healthcare leadership in the UK and Ireland requires navigating complex systems shaped by historical legacy, political priorities, regulatory structures, workforce pressures, economic constraints, and accelerating innovation. Leaders who understand this landscape are better equipped to make strategic decisions, build partnerships, manage risks, and drive meaningful change.

The chapters that follow build on this foundation by providing practical tools and leadership principles for managing teams, improving quality, leading change, and shaping the future of healthcare across these two interconnected systems.

CHAPTER 2

The Role of Management in Healthcare

Effective management is the backbone of healthcare delivery in the UK and Ireland. While leadership focuses on vision, culture, and influence, management ensures the systems, processes, resources, and people required for high-quality care are aligned and functioning. Both are essential, and both must work in tandem.

This chapter clarifies the purpose of healthcare management, outlines the competencies required in modern health systems, and explores the unique ethical responsibilities that come with managing services that directly affect people's lives.

2.1 Defining Healthcare Management in the UK and Ireland

Healthcare management is distinct from general management because it operates within systems that are:

- Safety-critical
- Resource-constrained
- Highly regulated
- Politically sensitive
- Multidisciplinary
- Value-driven (quality, dignity, fairness, equity)

It involves coordinating people, information, processes, and partnerships to ensure that care is safe, effective, person-centred, and sustainable.

2.1.1 The UK Context

Healthcare managers in the NHS work within organisational structures such as Acute Trusts, Mental Health Trusts, Community Trusts, and Integrated Care Systems (ICSs). They must balance:

- National targets and regulatory requirements
- Local population needs
- Workforce pressures
- Financial performance
- Governance, risk, and quality outcomes
- Digital transformation agendas
- Partnership working across health and social care

Modern NHS management places strong emphasis on:

- System leadership
- Quality improvement
- Workforce engagement
- Performance accountability
- Equity and population health

Managers are required to navigate political influence, complex commissioning environments, and increasing public scrutiny.

2.1.2 The Irish Context

Managers within the HSE and voluntary hospital system face similar but distinct demands. Irish healthcare managers must address:

- Sláintecare reform implementation
- Access and waiting list pressures
- Integration of health and social care
- Workforce shortages across primary, community, and acute care
- National clinical programmes
- HIQA standards and inspections
- Increasing expectations for transparency and service-user engagement

Unlike the NHS, Ireland's system includes a significant voluntary provider sector, requiring managers to build strong inter-organisational relationships and coordinate across governance structures.

Both systems demand managers who are skilled at strategic planning, operational oversight, financial management, quality assurance, and change leadership.

2.2 Managerial Skills and Competencies

Modern healthcare managers require a portfolio of technical, interpersonal, and behavioural competencies. These skills are not optional they are essential for success.

Below is a practical model used widely across the UK & Ireland:

2.2.1 Leadership and Behavioural Competence

While "leaders lead" and "managers manage," the most effective healthcare managers blend both sets of behaviours. Core behavioural competencies include:

• Setting clear expectations and holding people accountable
• Managing performance fairly and consistently
• Building psychologically safe team environments

- Influencing across professional boundaries
- Modelling integrity, equity, and compassion
- Remaining calm and effective under pressure
- Making evidence-informed decisions
- Engaging staff in change rather than imposing it

Behavioural competence often determines managerial effectiveness more than technical knowledge.

2.2.2 Financial and Resource Management

Healthcare managers must balance quality with affordability. This requires:

- Understanding budgets, cost pressures, and service demand
- Workforce planning and skill mix optimisation
- Prioritising investments based on value and risk
- Using data to identify inefficiencies
- Managing agency and overtime costs
- Ensuring services meet financial governance standards

In modern healthcare, financial awareness is not the job of finance departments alone **it is a fundamental part of operational and clinical management**.

2.2.3 Strategic Thinking and Planning

Managers must be capable of:

• Analysing trends (demographic, technological, policy, workforce)
• Setting SMART, measurable, system-aligned objectives
• Aligning local plans with national strategies (e.g., Sláintecare, NHS Long Term Plan)
• Conducting SWOT and PESTLE assessments
• Designing service improvements based on need, not habit
• Identifying risks and mitigation strategies
• Translating strategy into day-to-day operations

Effective managers see beyond immediate pressures and work with a horizon of 12–36 months.

2.2.4 Communication and Interpersonal Skills

Healthcare is relational. Managers must:

• Communicate clearly, directly, and consistently
• Give constructive feedback and manage difficult conversations
• Listen actively and empathetically
• Present confidently to staff and senior leaders
• Write reports that are accurate, structured, and actionable

• Build trust across disciplines, unions, and external partners
• Handle conflict professionally and fairly

A manager's ability to communicate will often define how their decisions are received.

2.2.5 Data Literacy and Quality Improvement

The ability to understand and use data is fundamental to modern healthcare management.

Managers must be skilled at:

• Reading dashboards and interpreting trends
• Understanding quality and safety indicators
• Using audit, benchmarking, and outcome measurement
• Supporting incident reviews and learning systems
• Applying QI methodologies (PDSA cycles, Lean, Six Sigma fundamentals)
• Turning data into meaningful improvement actions

Data-driven decision-making is now a core expectation, not an advanced skill.

2.3 Ethical Responsibilities in Healthcare Management

Healthcare managers carry significant ethical responsibility because their decisions directly influence patient care, staff well-being, and public trust.

2.3.1 Patient Confidentiality and Data Protection

Managers must ensure:

- GDPR compliance (Ireland & UK)
- Secure information systems
- Clear governance for access to patient records
- Staff training on confidentiality obligations
- Transparent processes for reporting breaches

Confidentiality failures damage trust and can cause harm.

2.3.2 Informed Consent and Patient Autonomy

While clinicians lead consent processes, managers must ensure:

- Policies and training are in place
- Systems support shared decision-making
- Patients receive clear, understandable information
- Cultural and language needs are respected

Patient-centred care requires organisational support, not just clinician skill.

2.3.3 Equity and Access to Care

Managers must actively challenge:

• Inequitable service provision
• Barriers created by geography, disability, language, or socioeconomic status
• Disparities in waiting times
• Bias in care pathways

Leadership in both countries increasingly demands a focus on **reducing health inequalities**.

2.3.4 Ethical Decision-Making in Resource-Limited Environments

Managers frequently face dilemmas involving:

• Competing priorities
• Limited capacity
• Workforce shortages
• Financial constraints
• Balancing organisational vs. patient benefit

Ethical frameworks help managers make transparent, defensible decisions that align with values such as justice, fairness, and beneficence.

Conclusion

Healthcare management in the UK and Ireland requires far more than operational oversight. Managers are strategic partners, culture shapers, system navigators, and ethical stewards. Their actions influence quality, safety, workforce morale, population outcomes, and organisational reputation.

Strong management is a critical pillar of effective healthcare leadership. As systems evolve, managers at all levels must cultivate the skills, behaviours, and ethical foundations required to deliver high-quality care in increasingly complex environments.

CHAPTER 3

Strategic Planning and Decision-Making

Strategic planning and decision-making are central responsibilities for healthcare managers and leaders. In environments where resources are constrained, demand is rising, and operational pressures are relentless, the ability to think clearly, plan effectively, and make informed decisions distinguishes high-performing services from struggling ones.

This chapter explores practical strategic planning processes, system-aligned goal-setting, evidence-based decision-making models, and the critical leadership role in risk and patient safety management across the UK and Ireland.

3.1 Developing a Strategic Plan for Healthcare Organisations

Strategic planning provides direction, clarity, and coherence. In healthcare where services must operate safely, efficiently, compassionately, and within regulatory frameworks it is essential.

A strong strategic plan answers four foundational questions:

1. **Where are we now?** (current state assessment)

2. **Where do we need to be?** (vision and future state)

3. **How will we get there?** (strategic initiatives)

4. **How will we know we're making progress?** (measurement and evaluation)

Below is a practical strategic planning model widely used across both systems.

3.1.1 Environmental Analysis (Understanding Context)

Healthcare leaders must understand the internal and external forces shaping their services. A structured analysis such as PESTLE or SWOT helps identify:

PESTLE Factors

• **Political:** NHS reforms, Sláintecare implementation, HIQA standards, regulatory pressure
• **Economic:** Budgets, workforce costs, inflation, efficiency targets
• **Social:** Ageing populations, health inequalities, cultural diversity, service-user expectations
• **Technological:** Digital health, virtual consultations, AI, data infrastructure
• **Legal:** GDPR, safeguarding, clinical governance, employment law
• **Environmental:** Infection prevention, sustainability, climate resilience

Environmental scanning is not a one-off exercise it requires continuous monitoring.

Internal Assessment

Leaders should analyse:
• Workforce capability and morale
• Capacity, demand, and throughput
• Performance metrics and quality outcomes

- Infrastructure, equipment, and IT systems
- Financial pressures and opportunities

Strategic plans must be grounded in reality, not aspiration.

3.1.2 Mission, Vision, and Values

A credible organisational strategy is rooted in clarity of purpose.

Mission

Defines *why* the organisation exists.
Example:
"To deliver safe, evidence-based, person-centred care that meets the needs of our communities."

Vision

Describes *what the organisation aspires to become*.
Example:
"To be a high-performing, innovative service recognised for excellence, equity, and compassion."

Values

Anchor behaviour and culture:
- Integrity
- Respect
- Compassion
- Accountability
- Learning

Leaders are responsible for ensuring that mission, vision, and values inform all strategic decisions, not simply appear on posters.

3.1.3 Goal Setting: SMART, System-Aligned Objectives

Healthcare goals must be meaningful, measurable, and directly connected to system priorities such as:

UK Examples

- NHS Long Term Plan objectives
- Integrated Care System (ICS) priorities
- CQC quality expectations
- Trust-level performance goals

Ireland Examples

- Sláintecare principles
- HSE National Service Plan objectives
- HIQA standards and improvement recommendations
- National Clinical Programmes

SMART Goals

Effective goals are:
Specific
Measurable
Achievable
Relevant
Time-bound

Example:
"Reduce elective surgery waiting times by 15% within 12 months through pathway redesign, enhanced triage, and improved scheduling systems."

3.1.4 Strategic Initiatives and Implementation

A goal without a plan remains a concept. Implementation requires:

Clear strategic initiatives, such as:

• Redesigning care pathways
• Improving digital integration
• Enhancing workforce wellbeing
• Expanding community-based care
• Strengthening quality governance

Operational Action Plans should define:

• Who is responsible
• What resources are needed
• Key milestones
• Dependencies
• Anticipated risks and mitigation
• Metrics for evaluation

Implementation succeeds when managers ensure ownership, accountability, and regular review.

3.2 Setting Goals and Objectives in the UK and Ireland Context

Because both systems have national priorities, local objectives must align with wider strategy.

3.2.1 In the UK

Healthcare organisations must show alignment with:

- **ICS population health priorities**
- **NHS England quality, access, and performance targets**
- **CQC Key Lines of Enquiry (KLOEs)**
- **Trust-level strategy and financial plans**

Examples of UK-aligned objectives:

- Improve A&E 4-hour performance through new streaming and triage processes
- Reduce outpatient backlog using virtual consultation pathways
- Strengthen safeguarding compliance to 100% within six months
- Enhance staff engagement scores through targeted leadership development

---

3.2.2 In Ireland

Objectives must reflect national reform direction and regulatory expectations.

Alignment includes:

• Sláintecare's emphasis on integrated, community-based care
• HSE performance indicators (KPIs)
• HIQA inspection findings and compliance frameworks
• National clinical programmes (e.g., chronic disease management)

Examples:

• Establish a community diagnostics hub to reduce acute demand
• Implement HIQA audit recommendations within 90 days
• Improve mental health service capacity through expanded multidisciplinary teams
• Develop integrated pathways to reduce emergency admissions for older adults

---

3.3 Decision-Making Models and Approaches

Effective decision-making requires structure, transparency, and awareness of bias. Healthcare decisions often involve complexity, competing priorities, and ethical implications.

Below are practical models leaders can use:

3.3.1 Rational Decision-Making Model

A systematic approach involving:

1. Define the problem
2. Gather relevant information
3. Identify options
4. Evaluate options (risk, cost, impact, feasibility)
5. Make a decision
6. Implement
7. Review outcomes

Strengths: logical, evidence-driven, transparent
Limitations: slower; not ideal in crisis situations

3.3.2 Intuitive Decision-Making

Experienced leaders often draw on tacit knowledge and pattern recognition.

Appropriate when:
- Time is limited
- Situations are familiar
- Rapid action is required

But should be balanced with data and consultation.

3.3.3 Shared Decision-Making

Used when decisions affect multiple stakeholders. It enhances:

• Engagement
• Ownership
• Cultural buy-in
• Implementation success

Examples:
• Workforce redesign
• Service reconfiguration
• Clinical pathway changes
• Scheduling or rota improvements

Shared decision-making is a sign of strong leadership—not weakness.

3.3.4 Ethical Decision-Making Frameworks

Healthcare decisions must be based on principles such as:

• Beneficence (doing good)
• Non-maleficence (avoiding harm)
• Justice (fairness)
• Autonomy (respecting choice)

Typical ethical decision steps:

1. Define the dilemma

2. Identify stakeholders

3. Consider ethical principles

4. Assess harms, benefits, and fairness

5. Explore alternatives

6. Make a transparent, defensible decision

This framework is especially useful for decisions involving constrained resources or service prioritisation.

3.4 Risk Management and Patient Safety in the UK and Ireland

Risk and patient safety are core responsibilities of healthcare managers. Failures in this area can have catastrophic consequences clinically, legally, and reputationally.

3.4.1 The UK Approach

Key components include:

- National Patient Safety Strategy
- Duty of Candour
- Learning from patient safety incidents (LFPSE)
- CQC regulations
- Trust-level risk registers

- Morbidity and mortality reviews
- Datix/incident reporting systems

Managers must:

- Encourage transparent reporting
- Ensure timely incident investigations
- Track trends and emerging risks
- Provide feedback and learning loops
- Embed a just culture

3.4.2 The Irish Approach

Key elements include:

- National Incident Management System (NIMS)
- HIQA standards and inspections
- Serious Incident Management Team (SIMT) processes
- National Clinical Programmes for quality and safety
- Clinical audit and risk registers
- Open Disclosure Policy

Managers must support teams by:

- Ensuring staff training in risk management
- Responding appropriately to incidents
- Implementing corrective actions
- Monitoring compliance
- Communicating learning across teams

Conclusion

Strategic planning and decision-making are not theoretical exercises they shape the daily realities of staff, patients, and communities. Leaders who understand their context, assess risk, use data effectively, and make thoughtful decisions are better equipped to:

- Improve quality
- Strengthen performance
- Deliver safer, more reliable services
- Build trust across teams
- Navigate political and organisational pressures

With a clear strategy and robust decision-making framework, healthcare organisations can remain resilient even in the face of significant system pressures.

CHAPTER 4

Organisational Design and Structure

Organisational design is central to effective healthcare leadership. The way a service is structured its teams, decision-making pathways, communication flows, and accountability systems determines its ability to deliver safe, high-quality, efficient, patient-centred care. Good people cannot overcome poor system design;

therefore leaders must understand how structure impacts behaviour, performance, culture, and outcomes.

This chapter examines the principles of effective organisational design, the role of team-based care, how to cultivate a collaborative culture, and the challenges of leading change in the complex healthcare systems of the UK and Ireland.

4.1 Designing Effective Healthcare Organisations in the UK and Ireland

Effective organisational design ensures that the right people, processes, and systems are connected in a way that supports clear communication, efficient workflow, and accountability. In healthcare, the design must balance clinical priorities, regulatory requirements, safety, workforce needs, and financial constraints.

Core principles of strong organisational design:

• Alignment with strategy and patient needs
• Clear roles and decision-making authority
• Effective communication channels
• Staff empowerment and team cohesion
• Integration across pathways and services
• Responsiveness to system demands and risk
• Built-in mechanisms for learning and improvement

Both the NHS and the HSE have undergone significant restructuring to adapt to population growth, rising demand, workforce challenges, and the shift towards integrated care.

4.1.1 Structural Considerations

Healthcare organisations typically adopt one or a combination of the following structures:

Hierarchical Structures

Traditional, top-down models with clear authority and reporting lines.
Strengths: clarity, stability, regulatory compliance.
Weaknesses: risk of silos, slow decision-making.

Common in acute hospitals and large Trusts/HSE directorates.

Matrix Structures

Staff may report to multiple managers (e.g., clinical lead + operational manager).
Strengths: flexibility, resource optimisation, interdisciplinary collaboration.
Challenges: role confusion, conflict over priorities.

Increasingly used in clinical directorates and multidisciplinary pathways.

Networked/Integrated Care Structures

Teams and organisations form networks across health, mental health, social care, community, and voluntary sectors.

Examples:
• Integrated Care Systems (ICSs) in England
• Sláintecare Community Healthcare Networks in Ireland

Strengths: patient-centred, holistic, reduces fragmentation.
Challenges: diffuse accountability, complex governance.

Lean or Value-Stream Structures

Designed around patient flow rather than departments.
Example: structured pathways for stroke, cancer, maternity, chronic disease.

Strengths: efficiency, reduced delays, improved outcomes.
Challenges: requires cultural change and redesign of long-standing practices.

4.1.2 Governance and Leadership

Strong governance ensures that organisations meet their responsibility for safety, quality, financial control, and compliance.

Key governance elements include:

• Clear lines of accountability from frontline to board/executive
• Well-defined clinical governance processes
• Robust risk and incident management systems
• Regular quality audits, dashboards, and performance reports
• Visible leadership behaviours that model integrity and transparency

In the UK:

Trust Boards, ICS Governance, CQC frameworks, and NHS England oversight all shape organisational accountability.

In Ireland:

HSE structures, voluntary hospital boards, HIQA standards, Mental Health Commission oversight, and Sláintecare reforms form the governance landscape.

Effective governance is not about bureaucracy it is about ensuring safety, learning, and responsible stewardship.

4.1.3 Workforce Planning and Human Resources

Workforce is the most critical asset in healthcare. Organisational design must ensure:

- Appropriate staffing levels
- Skill mix optimisation
- Fair and manageable workloads
- Opportunities for career progression
- Psychological safety and wellbeing support
- Recruitment, induction, and retention strategies
- Leadership development and talent pipelines

Workforce shortages across both countries make planning more important than ever. Leaders must use data, scenario modelling, and proactive engagement to stabilise services.

4.2 Team-Based Approaches in Healthcare

Team-based care is essential for delivering safe, effective, integrated services. Healthcare has moved far beyond the single-discipline model; success now depends on collaboration across professions, departments, and sectors.

4.2.1 Interprofessional Teams

Interprofessional teams bring together different disciplines to deliver coordinated care.

Common examples include:

- Medical, nursing, and allied health teams
- Community health and social care partnerships
- Mental health multidisciplinary teams
- Integrated chronic disease management teams

Benefits:

- Improved patient outcomes
- Reduced duplication and error
- Better communication and handovers
- Enhanced staff satisfaction
- Shared accountability

Leaders must ensure these teams have clear goals, defined roles, and structured communication processes (e.g., MDT meetings, handover tools).

4.2.2 Multidisciplinary Teams (MDTs)

MDTs focus on complex patient needs and are essential in areas like oncology, stroke, mental health, and paediatrics.

Effective MDTs require:
- Shared decision-making
- Rapid information exchange
- Respect for diverse expertise
- Clear, documented care plans

A poorly coordinated MDT can introduce risk; strong leadership and structure are therefore essential.

4.2.3 Patient Engagement as Part of the Team

Patient-centred systems treat patients and families as active contributors.

This includes:
• Shared decision-making
• Self-management support
• Co-design of pathways
• Accessible information
• Cultural and linguistic support

Services that engage patients meaningfully see higher satisfaction, fewer complaints, and improved outcomes.

4.3 Creating a Culture of Collaboration

Structures matter, but *culture determines behaviour.* A collaborative culture encourages teamwork, innovation, transparency, and psychological safety.

4.3.1 Communication and Information Sharing

Healthcare requires constant, precise communication.

Leaders should ensure:

• Use of standardised tools (SBAR, structured handovers)
• Effective digital communication systems
• Timely dissemination of policies, updates, and decisions
• Regular team meetings with clear purposes
• Feedback loops for learning and improvement

Communication failures are among the highest contributors to patient safety incidents.

4.3.2 Leadership That Enables Collaboration

Collaborative cultures depend on leaders who:

• Are visible and approachable
• Value staff input
• Address concerns early
• Give recognition generously
• Promote shared goals over personal agendas
• Resolve conflict fairly and objectively
• Encourage learning, not blame

Leaders set the tone for how teams behave.

4.3.3 Collaboration Tools and Technologies

Digital tools that support collaboration include:

- Shared electronic health records
- MDT virtual meeting platforms
- Document-sharing systems
- Digital whiteboards for patient flow
- Real-time data dashboards

However, technology must be introduced with training, consultation, and clear purpose.

4.4 Managing Change in the UK and Ireland Healthcare Systems

Change is constant in healthcare whether driven by policy, demand, workforce issues, new technology, or quality concerns. Leaders must be skilled at facilitating change in a way that is structured, compassionate, and sustainable.

4.4.1 Understanding the Change Process

Widely used frameworks include:

Kotter's 8-Step Change Model

1. Establish urgency

2. Build a guiding coalition

3. Form a vision

4. Communicate the vision

5. Remove obstacles

6. Generate short-term wins

7. Sustain acceleration

8. Anchor changes in culture

ADKAR Model (Individual-Level Change)

Awareness → Desire → Knowledge → Ability → Reinforcement

Change fails when leaders underestimate the emotional and behavioural components.

4.4.2 Stakeholder Engagement

Healthcare leaders must bring people with them not push them forward.

Effective engagement includes:

- Early involvement
- Active listening
- Acknowledging concerns
- Clear explanation of benefits
- Co-designing solutions
- Regular updates
- Celebrating progress

When stakeholders feel valued, resistance decreases and ownership increases.

4.4.3 Change Communication

Clear, consistent, honest communication is essential.

Leaders should communicate:

- Why change is needed
- What the change involves
- How it affects staff
- How risks will be managed
- Timeframes and expectations
- Support available
- Progress and outcomes

Silence creates speculation; speculation creates resistance.

Conclusion

Organisational design shapes the conditions in which staff work and patients receive care. Effective structures, strong governance, collaborative teams, and well-managed change processes enable safe, high-quality, person-centred healthcare.

Healthcare organisations in the UK and Ireland are evolving rapidly. Leaders who understand organisational dynamics and who invest in communication, culture, teamwork, and change will be best positioned to deliver services that are resilient, compassionate, and future-ready.

CHAPTER 5

Human Resource Management

The workforce is the beating heart of every healthcare organisation. No strategy, technology, or clinical innovation can succeed without a skilled, motivated, healthy, and supported workforce. Yet healthcare systems across the UK and Ireland face unprecedented challenges: staffing shortages, recruitment difficulties, burnout, rising demand, high turnover, and increased expectations from staff and patients.

Effective Human Resource Management (HRM) is therefore one of the most critical leadership responsibilities in modern healthcare. HRM must extend far beyond transactional tasks it must actively shape culture, support wellbeing, develop talent, and build an environment where staff feel valued and able to deliver safe, high-quality care.

This chapter provides practical guidance for today's healthcare leaders on recruitment, engagement, performance, development, and retention.

5.1 Recruitment and Selection in the UK and Ireland Healthcare Sector

Recruiting staff in modern healthcare is a strategic activity, not an administrative function. Leaders must anticipate needs, plan proactively, and compete for talent in a highly mobile, international workforce.

5.1.1 Workforce Planning and Forecasting

Good recruitment starts with understanding future workforce needs.

Leaders should analyse:

• Demand projections (e.g., ageing population, chronic disease management, service expansion)
• Workforce supply (retirements, turnover, vacancies, specialist shortages)
• Skill mix and role redesign opportunities (advanced nurse practitioners, assistant practitioners, integrated care roles)
• Organisational growth or restructuring plans
• National shortages in nursing, general practice, social care, mental health, and allied health professions

Workforce planning helps organisations avoid crisis-driven recruitment and ensures services can operate safely and sustainably.

5.1.2 Attracting and Sourcing Talent

Both the NHS and HSE face fierce competition for staff. Leaders must therefore build an employer brand that appeals to modern professionals.

Key strategies include:

• Clear messaging about organisational values and culture
• Flexible work options (particularly post-pandemic)
• Career progression pathways
• Training and development opportunities
• Attractive wellbeing supports
• Strong reputation for quality and safety
• Inclusion, equity, and diversity initiatives
• Effective use of social media, job boards, and professional networks
• International recruitment where appropriate

A positive reputation is one of the most powerful recruitment assets.

5.1.3 Selection and Assessment

Healthcare requires staff with technical competence *and* emotional intelligence. Selection processes should therefore combine:

• Structured interviews
• Scenario-based assessments

- Values-based recruitment tools
- Professional competency checks
- Background and reference verification
- Practical or clinical assessments where appropriate

Values-based recruitment (VBR) is increasingly used to ensure alignment with organisational culture, compassion, teamwork, and patient-centred care.

5.2 Employee Engagement and Motivation in Healthcare Settings

Engaged staff perform better, stay longer, innovate more, and contribute to safer care. Engagement is shaped less by pay or workload and more by **leadership behaviour**, **culture**, **autonomy**, and **recognition**.

5.2.1 Creating a Supportive Organisational Culture

Culture determines how people feel, behave, and perform at work.

A supportive culture requires:

- Psychological safety staff feel comfortable speaking up
- Clear communication and transparent decision-making
- Recognition and appreciation

- Team cohesion and mutual respect
- Learning rather than blame
- Fair and consistent leadership
- Inclusion and belonging

Leaders shape culture through their everyday actions.

5.2.2 Effective Leadership and Management Practices

Motivation is directly linked to the quality of local management.

Effective leaders:

- Give clear expectations
- Provide regular, constructive feedback
- Address issues early and fairly
- Celebrate success
- Welcome staff ideas and improvement suggestions
- Allocate workload realistically
- Show empathy, presence, and support during pressures
- Protect staff wellbeing and boundaries
- Are accessible and approachable

Leadership behaviour is one of the strongest predictors of workforce retention.

5.2.3 Work-Life Balance and Wellbeing

Healthcare work is emotionally demanding and high-risk. If wellbeing is neglected, service quality declines.

Leaders must ensure:

- Flexible and predictable rosters where possible
- Access to mental health and employee assistance programmes
- Peer support systems
- Debriefing following traumatic events
- Support for return-to-work processes
- Fair management of annual leave and breaks
- Initiatives to address burnout (mindfulness sessions, mentoring, workload reviews)

A healthy workforce is essential for safe patient care.

5.3 Performance Management and Evaluation in the UK and Ireland

Performance management is not about policing staff it is about supporting development, maintaining standards, and ensuring safe, reliable care.

5.3.1 Performance Expectations and Goal Setting

Performance must be linked to:

• Organisational strategy (e.g., ICS goals, Sláintecare KPIs)
• Quality and safety standards
• Professional standards and codes of practice
• Individual role clarity

Effective leaders set goals that are:

• Clear
• Collaborative
• Achievable
• Outcome-focused

When expectations are unclear, performance suffers.

5.3.2 Performance Feedback and Coaching

Feedback is most effective when it is:

• Timely
• Specific
• Balanced
• Respectful
• Linked to behaviour and impact
• Future- rather than past-focused

Coaching improves:

• Confidence
• Skill development
• Insight

- Motivation
- Problem-solving

Coaching conversations should be routine not reserved for difficulties.

5.3.3 Performance Recognition and Rewards

Recognition is a powerful motivator.

Examples include:

- Public acknowledgement
- Nomination for awards
- Opportunities to lead projects
- Funded training or CPD
- Written appreciation from senior leaders
- Peer-recognition programmes

Recognition should be frequent, genuine, and aligned with organisational values.

5.4 Training and Development of Healthcare Professionals

Learning is essential in a constantly evolving sector. Healthcare staff must stay current with clinical advances, legislation, digital systems, and quality standards.

5.4.1 Continuing Education and Professional Development

Leaders must provide access to:

• Formal training (courses, diplomas, postgraduate qualifications)
• Mandatory training (safeguarding, infection prevention, GDPR)
• E-learning modules
• Simulation training
• Multi-disciplinary workshops
• Conferences and professional networks

A learning-rich environment is a retention strategy in itself.

5.4.2 Leadership Development

Future-proofing the workforce requires investment in leadership.

Organisations should provide:

• Leadership programmes for all stages emerging, experienced, and senior leaders
• Coaching and mentoring
• Shadowing and secondment opportunities
• Training in emotional intelligence, communication, conflict resolution, and systems leadership

Strong leadership capacity is critical for sustaining organisational performance.

5.4.3 Technology Training and Digital Literacy

Digital transformation requires digitally confident staff.

Training should cover:

- Electronic patient records
- Virtual care systems
- AI-supported clinical tools
- Data dashboards and reporting
- Cybersecurity awareness
- Interoperability and information-sharing pathways

Digital competence improves efficiency, safety, and staff confidence.

5.5 Retaining and Developing Talent in the UK and Ireland Healthcare Systems

Retention is now one of the most pressing workforce challenges. Leaders must create workplaces where people want to stay and feel they can grow.

5.5.1 Talent Management and Succession Planning

Identify high-potential staff early and invest in them.

Key tasks include:

- Mapping critical roles and future vacancies
- Developing internal talent pipelines
- Providing targeted development opportunities
- Formal succession plans for senior roles
- Encouraging cross-departmental mobility

A stable leadership pipeline improves organisational resilience.

5.5.2 Workforce Diversity and Inclusion

Inclusive organisations are more innovative, perform better, and retain staff more effectively.

Leaders must ensure:

- Recruitment processes free from bias
- Diverse interview panels
- Accessible career progression
- Anti-racism and anti-discrimination policies
- Support networks for minority groups
- Respect for cultural and personal identity
- Psychological safety for all staff

Diversity strengthens decision-making and patient care.

5.5.3 Workforce Wellbeing, Burnout Prevention, and Work-Life Balance

Burnout is a patient safety issue. It reduces concentration, compassion, productivity, and retention.

To prevent burnout, leaders must:

• Monitor workload intensity
• Encourage regular breaks
• Address toxic behaviours swiftly
• Ensure safe staffing levels
• Promote realistic expectations
• Provide wellbeing supports
• Model healthy habits themselves

Healthy staff deliver healthier care.

Conclusion

Human Resource Management in healthcare is about far more than hiring staff and maintaining records. It is about cultivating a workforce that is skilled, supported, engaged, and resilient. Leaders who invest in staff wellbeing, recognise contribution, support development, and create a safe, inclusive culture are the ones who build high-performing, sustainable services.

The challenges in the UK and Ireland are significant workforce shortages, rising demand, burnout, and recruitment pressures but strong leadership can make the decisive difference.

A valued workforce becomes a committed workforce, and a committed workforce becomes the foundation of safe, high-quality healthcare.

CHAPTER 6

The Essence of Leadership in Healthcare

Leadership in healthcare is unlike leadership in any other sector. The work is emotionally demanding, politically sensitive, safety-critical, highly regulated, multidisciplinary, and deeply human. Leaders must balance compassion with accountability, strategy with operational pressure, and ambition with limited resources. They must influence across boundaries, navigate system complexity, and inspire staff who are often under extreme strain.

This chapter explores what leadership *really* means in today's NHS, HSE, and wider health and social care systems. It examines leadership styles, emotional intelligence, the importance of role modelling, and the central role of trust and credibility in shaping organisational culture.

6.1 Leadership Styles and Approaches in the UK and Ireland

No single leadership style meets the needs of every situation. Effective healthcare leaders are versatile they adapt their approach to context, team readiness, organisational culture, and the urgency of the challenges they face.

Below are the leadership styles most relevant to modern healthcare.

6.1.1 Transformational Leadership

Transformational leaders inspire, motivate, and elevate performance by:

- Creating a compelling vision
- Communicating purpose clearly and passionately
- Supporting innovation and creativity
- Empowering staff to take ownership
- Building strong relationships
- Encouraging continuous learning
- Fostering a positive, inclusive culture

Transformational leadership is linked to higher staff morale, reduced burnout, improved patient outcomes, and stronger team cohesion. It is considered one of the most effective styles in healthcare.

Example:
A director of nursing introduces a shared governance model, enabling nurses to influence policy, improve

practice, and lead quality initiatives. Staff feel valued, morale improves, and care becomes more consistent.

6.1.2 Transactional Leadership

This approach focuses on structure, tasks, and performance.

- Clear expectations
- Defined duties
- Rewards and consequences
- Monitoring for compliance

While sometimes criticised as rigid, transactional leadership is essential for:

- Maintaining safety
- Meeting regulatory requirements
- Managing high-risk environments
- Ensuring policies and protocols are followed

Most healthcare leaders use a blend of transformational and transactional behaviours.

6.1.3 Distributed (Shared) Leadership

In distributed leadership, influence is shared across roles, teams, and levels not held solely by those in formal positions.

It is particularly effective in:

- Integrated care
- Multidisciplinary teams
- Quality improvement projects
- Clinical leadership development
- Large, complex hospital systems

Distributed leadership improves engagement, innovation, and ownership because staff feel part of the solution not subjects of top-down change.

Example:
A hospital introduces ward-based improvement teams led by frontline staff, who redesign care processes with support from management.

6.1.4 Situational Leadership

Situational leadership adapts style to the readiness and capability of the individual or team.

This is essential in healthcare, where teams vary in experience, confidence, and maturity. A leader may need to:

- Direct and support a newly formed team
- Delegate to an expert group
- Coach a developing clinician
- Collaborate with a senior multidisciplinary team

The most effective leaders are agile they adapt quickly to what their staff need.

6.2 Emotional Intelligence and Leadership in Healthcare Settings

Emotional Intelligence (EI) is one of the strongest predictors of leadership effectiveness in healthcare. Leaders who lack EI struggle with communication, conflict, staff engagement, and team morale.

EI involves four key domains:

6.2.1 Self-Awareness

Leaders must understand their:

- Emotions
- Strengths and limitations
- Stress triggers
- Behavioural patterns
- Impact on others

Self-aware leaders demonstrate humility, accept feedback, and regulate their emotional responses.

Example:
Recognising when frustration may affect tone, a leader takes a moment to reset before addressing a team concern.

6.2.2 Self-Management

This includes:

- Emotional regulation
- Resilience under pressure
- Adaptability
- Calm decision-making
- Maintaining professionalism in difficult moments

Healthcare is unpredictable; leaders must remain composed even in complex or high-risk situations.

6.2.3 Social Awareness

This involves:

- Empathy
- Understanding team needs
- Acknowledging stress, workload, and emotional impact
- Cultural sensitivity
- Recognition of power dynamics

Leaders with strong social awareness pick up subtle cues that others may miss, enabling them to prevent escalation and support their teams effectively.

6.2.4 Relationship Management

High-quality relationships enable:

• Trust
• Collaboration
• Conflict resolution
• Motivation
• Team cohesion
• Honest communication

Leaders who invest in relationships build psychologically safe teams where staff feel able to speak up, innovate, and challenge unsafe practices.

6.3 Leading by Example: The Power of Role Modelling

Healthcare leaders are watched more closely than they realise. Their behaviour positive or negative becomes a signal of what is acceptable.

Leading by example means:

• Demonstrating professionalism consistently
• Making ethically sound decisions
• Communicating respectfully
• Being visible, approachable, and engaged
• Taking responsibility for mistakes
• Showing genuine compassion
• Following policies they expect others to follow
• Role-modelling work-life balance and wellbeing

The behaviours leaders demonstrate shape organisational culture more powerfully than any strategy document.

6.3.1 Professionalism and Ethical Behaviour

Patients, families, regulators, and staff expect leaders to uphold the highest ethical standards.

Ethical leadership requires:

- Honesty
- Fairness
- Accountability
- Transparency
- Respect for dignity
- Appropriate boundaries
- Avoidance of blame culture

Ethical lapses destroy trust quickly and trust is the currency of healthcare leadership.

6.3.2 Commitment to Continuous Learning

Healthcare is evolving rapidly. Leaders must model lifelong learning by:

- Updating knowledge
- Completing leadership training
- Seeking feedback
- Reflecting on performance

• Staying informed about clinical and policy developments

A leader who stops learning stops leading.

6.4 Building Trust and Credibility in Healthcare Leadership

Trust is the foundation of every successful team. Without it, staff disengage, communication breaks down, and organisational culture deteriorates.

Healthcare leaders build trust through consistent behaviour over time.

6.4.1 Open and Transparent Communication

Staff trust leaders who:

• Communicate honestly
• Share important information promptly
• Listen actively
• Explain decisions clearly
• Admit when they don't know something
• Discuss mistakes with humility

Transparency reduces anxiety and strengthens team cohesion.

6.4.2 Consistency and Reliability

Credibility comes from:

- Doing what you say you will do
- Treating people fairly and consistently
- Following through on commitments
- Making decisions based on evidence and values
- Staying calm and dependable in crisis situations

Consistency builds psychological safety staff know what to expect.

6.4.3 Empowerment and Delegation

Effective leaders:

- Delegate appropriately
- Encourage autonomy
- Trust staff to own their work
- Support innovation and initiative
- Provide guidance without micromanaging

Empowerment improves motivation, creativity, and capacity-building across the organisation.

Conclusion

Leadership in healthcare requires emotional intelligence, adaptability, compassion, decisiveness, and integrity. It demands a deep understanding of people, systems, culture, and context. Leaders must inspire, guide, and support staff in environments marked by constant change, complexity, and pressure.

Strong leadership is not defined by title or authority but by behaviour.

Leaders who build trust, communicate openly, demonstrate empathy, model ethical practice, and empower teams create the conditions for high-quality care and sustainable organisational resilience. As the UK and Ireland continue to reform their health systems, the need for skilled, compassionate, and credible leaders has never been greater.

CHAPTER 7

Effective Communication and Relationship Building

Communication is one of the most essential competencies for any healthcare leader. It influences safety, performance, trust, morale, and culture. Poor communication is a leading cause of patient harm, conflict, staff disengagement, and organisational failure. Conversely, clear, compassionate, and consistent communication strengthens relationships, builds credibility, and supports effective teamwork across complex systems.

This chapter explores the foundations of professional communication, the importance of active listening and empathy, strategies for conflict resolution, and the critical role of communication in building strong relationships within and across healthcare organisations.

7.1 Foundations of Effective Communication in Healthcare

Healthcare is fast-paced and high-risk. Messages must be accurate, structured, and timely. Leaders must be deliberate communicators who can adapt their style to suit the situation, audience, and environment.

7.1.1 Active Listening

Effective communication begins with listening not speaking. Active listening involves:

- Giving full attention
- Maintaining eye contact (where culturally appropriate)
- Avoiding interruption
- Reflecting or summarising to confirm understanding
- Acknowledging emotion without judgement
- Asking clarifying questions
- Demonstrating genuine interest

Active listening builds trust, prevents misunderstandings, and helps staff feel valued and understood.

Example:
A staff member expresses concern's about workload. Instead of offering quick solutions, the manager listens fully, validates their experience, and engages collaboratively in problem-solving.

7.1.2 Clarity and Precision in Messaging

Healthcare environments often involve stress, noise, time pressure, and complexity. Ambiguous communication can lead to serious consequences.

Clear communication requires:

• Simple, direct language
• Avoidance of jargon unless everyone understands it
• Structured frameworks (e.g., SBAR)
• Summarising key actions before closing a conversation
• Being specific about who is responsible for what
• Confirming understanding

Clarity prevents error and improves accountability.

7.1.3 Nonverbal Communication Cues

Nonverbal behaviour can reinforce or undermine verbal messages.

Important cues include:

- Facial expressions
- Body posture
- Tone of voice
- Level of attentiveness
- Positioning within a room
- Gestures
- Physical distance

Healthcare leaders must remain aware of how their presence affects staff, patients, and families.

7.2 Communication Tools and Technologies

Modern healthcare uses a combination of face-to-face communication and technology-supported systems. The challenge for leaders is to select the right channel for the right message.

7.2.1 Digital Communication Platforms

Tools commonly used in the UK and Ireland include:

- Secure email
- Intranet platforms

- Microsoft Teams / Zoom
- EHR communication notes
- Digital handover systems
- Task management tools
- Staff messaging systems

These tools improve efficiency but must be used thoughtfully.

7.2.2 Electronic Health Records (EHRs)

EHRs support:

- Information accuracy
- Continuity of care
- Shared access across professionals
- Better decision-making
- Reduced duplication

However, leaders must ensure staff have training, confidence, and time to use digital systems appropriately.

7.2.3 Telehealth and Virtual Care Platforms

Virtual communication requires adapted skills, especially when interacting with patients.

Leaders should ensure:

- Clear protocols for virtual consultations
- Training in remote communication skills
- Robust safeguarding procedures
- Confidential, secure platforms

Virtual care adds convenience but must not compromise safety, privacy, or rapport.

7.3 Interpersonal Communication in Healthcare Teams

Healthcare teams depend on trust, psychological safety, and shared goals. Effective interpersonal communication is foundational for collaborative practice.

7.3.1 Building Rapport and Trust

Rapport influences:

- Willingness to communicate openly
- Team cohesion
- Staff motivation
- Conflict resolution
- Engagement with organisational change

Strategies include:

• Being approachable and visible
• Showing appreciation
• Remembering personal details (e.g., interests, achievements)
• Being consistent in words and actions

Trust is built gradually through behaviour, not position.

7.3.2 Active Empathy and Emotional Intelligence

Empathy deepens understanding and reduces defensive reactions.

Empathic communication includes:

• Recognising emotional cues
• Validating feelings ("I can see why that was frustrating")
• Offering support without dismissing or minimising concerns
• Balancing compassion with clarity about boundaries

Empathy strengthens relationships and enhances staff wellbeing.

7.3.3 Managing Difficult Conversations

Difficult conversations are unavoidable. Leaders must address issues promptly, professionally, and respectfully.

Examples include:

• Performance concerns
• Behavioural issues
• Attendance problems
• Team conflict
• Safety concerns
• Feedback following incidents
• Sensitive or emotional situations

Effective strategies:

• Prepare ahead
• Focus on behaviour, not character
• Use neutral language
• Remain calm
• Allow the other person time to speak
• Agree clear next steps

Avoidance leads to greater conflict and poorer outcomes.

7.4 Conflict Resolution and Negotiation in Healthcare

Conflict is natural in multidisciplinary, high-pressure environments. Leaders must manage conflict early, objectively, and fairly.

7.4.1 Understanding the Sources of Conflict

Common causes include:

- Role ambiguity
- Resource constraints
- Differences in clinical opinion
- Communication breakdowns
- Personality clashes
- Stress, fatigue, and burnout
- Perceived unfairness
- Organisational change

Understanding the cause allows leaders to choose the right resolution strategy.

7.4.2 Mediation and Collaborative Problem-Solving

Effective conflict resolution requires:

- Establishing a safe, neutral space
- Encouraging both sides to express their perspective
- Identifying shared goals (e.g., patient safety)
- Focusing on solutions, not blame
- Clarifying expectations and agreements
- Documenting outcomes where needed

Leaders should remain impartial and respectful, modelling the behaviours expected during conflict.

7.4.3 Negotiation Strategies

In healthcare, negotiation occurs daily in staffing, resources, scheduling, interdepartmental collaboration, and system-level decision-making.

Effective negotiation involves:

- Preparation and clarity about objectives
- Understanding the other party's perspective
- Identifying non-negotiables vs. flexible areas
- Maintaining professionalism and respect
- Seeking mutually beneficial outcomes
- Focusing on shared priorities

Strong negotiation skills help leaders secure resources, resolve issues, and build collaborative partnerships.

7.5 Collaboration with Internal and External Stakeholders

Modern healthcare operates across boundaries. Leaders must communicate effectively with a wide range of stakeholders.

7.5.1 Internal Stakeholders

These include:

- Clinical teams (nursing, medical, AHPs)
- Administrative and operational staff
- Quality and safety teams
- HR, finance, and governance teams
- IT and digital health departments
- Senior management and board members

Communication must be:

- Tailored
- Respectful
- Transparent
- Timely
- Aligned with organisational strategy

7.5.2 External Stakeholders

Examples include:

- Regulators (HIQA, CQC, Mental Health Commission)
- Local authorities
- Voluntary and community organisations
- Patient advocacy groups
- Academic institutions
- Other health and social care providers
- Professional councils (GMC, NMBI, etc.)
- Media representatives

Leaders must protect organisational reputation by communicating:

- Accurately
- Professionally
- Sensitively
- In alignment with governance and communications policies

7.5.3 Building Multi-Agency Partnerships

Effective partnership working improves:

- Care coordination
- Service integration
- Patient outcomes
- Innovation
- Community health and wellbeing

Partnerships thrive when supported by:

- Clear communication channels
- Shared objectives
- Defined roles and responsibilities
- Trust and mutual respect

Conclusion

Communication and relationship building are essential leadership competencies.

Healthcare leaders do not work in isolation they operate within vast networks of staff, patients, families, teams, regulators, community partners, and multidisciplinary professionals.

Leaders who communicate clearly, listen actively, engage compassionately, resolve conflict fairly, and foster strong relationships build cultures where staff feel safe, valued, and connected to organisational purpose. These behaviours ultimately strengthen service quality, safety, and workforce resilience.

CHAPTER 8

Leading and Managing Change

Change is inevitable in healthcare. Systems evolve, policies shift, technologies advance, workforce needs fluctuate, and public expectations grow. Whether implementing digital systems, redesigning care pathways, responding to regulatory findings, or managing organisational reconfiguration, leaders must be skilled at guiding individuals and teams through change with clarity, compassion, and confidence.

This chapter explores the principles of effective change management, the psychological and behavioural responses to change, tools and models for implementation, and strategies for overcoming resistance.

It is written for leaders who must deliver change in the complex, regulated, emotionally charged environment of healthcare in the UK and Ireland.

8.1 Understanding the Need for Change in Healthcare

Change in healthcare is rarely optional. It is driven by internal and external forces that leaders must recognise and respond to.

8.1.1 Internal Drivers of Change

Examples include:

- Quality or safety concerns
- Staff shortages or skill mix pressures
- Financial deficits
- Operational inefficiencies
- Cultural or behavioural issues
- Poor patient experience
- Outdated processes or technology
- Strategic realignment

Internal change is often initiated to improve safety, performance, or sustainability.

8.1.2 External Drivers of Change

Key external influences include:

• National strategies (NHS Long Term Plan, Sláintecare)
• Regulation and inspection (CQC, HIQA, MHC)
• Legislation (GDPR, safeguarding, employment law)
• Demographic changes and rising demand
• Technological advances (AI, digital health, virtual care)
• Public expectation for transparency and patient-centred care
• Workforce challenges across both systems

Leaders must scan the horizon and anticipate change rather than react only when issues escalate.

8.2 Models of Change in Healthcare Leadership

Effective change requires structure. Below are two widely used models suitable for healthcare.

8.2.1 Lewin's Change Model

A simple but powerful framework:

1. Unfreeze

• Establish urgency
• Communicate clearly why change is necessary

- Challenge existing assumptions
- Prepare staff emotionally and practically

2. Change (Transition)

- Implement new processes or behaviours
- Provide training, support, and resources
- Encourage feedback
- Address concerns compassionately

3. Refreeze

- Embed new practices into policy and culture
- Monitor and reinforce behaviour
- Celebrate success and learning

Lewin's model emphasises the psychological element of change something healthcare leaders must never overlook.

8.2.2 Kotter's 8-Step Change Model

A more detailed, action-based model frequently used in organisational transformation:

1. **Create urgency**

2. **Build a guiding coalition**

3. **Form a strategic vision**

4. **Communicate the vision**

5. **Remove barriers**

6. **Generate short-term wins**

7. **Sustain momentum**

8. **Anchor change in organisational culture**

Kotter's model is ideal for large-scale change (e.g., digital transformation or service redesign).

8.3 Strategies for Successful Change Implementation

Leaders must combine technical planning with human understanding. Change succeeds or fails based on staff engagement, not simply process design.

8.3.1 Clear Vision and Communication

A compelling vision answers:

• What is changing?
• Why must it change?
• How will it work?
• What will be different for staff and patients?
• How will success be measured?

Communication should be:

• Continuous
• Honest
• Two-way
• Tailored to the audience

• Delivered through multiple channels (meetings, emails, workshops)

Silence creates uncertainty. Clarity builds trust.

8.3.2 Stakeholder Engagement Across Systems

Healthcare change affects many groups. Leaders must involve:

- Frontline staff
- Clinical leaders
- Operational managers
- Unions and professional bodies
- IT, HR, finance, and governance teams
- Patients and service users
- Community and voluntary partners
- Regulators, where appropriate

Engagement should begin early not once decisions have already been made.

8.3.3 Training and Capacity-Building

People resist what they do not understand or feel unprepared for.

Leaders should provide:

- Practical training
- Time to learn new systems

- Supervision and coaching
- Clear guidance documentation
- Peer support arrangements

Competence builds confidence; confidence reduces resistance.

8.3.4 Resource Allocation

Change without resources creates frustration and failure.

Resources may include:

- Staff time
- Equipment
- Technology
- Budget
- Dedicated project leads
- Protected learning time

Leaders must ensure resources match expectations.

8.3.5 Change Champions and Local Leadership

Identifying respected staff to act as "change champions" improves adoption and credibility.

Champions should:

- Model new behaviours
- Answer questions

- Support peers
- Escalate barriers
- Promote positivity and persistence

Peer-led influence is often more effective than senior instruction.

8.4 Overcoming Resistance to Change in Healthcare Teams

Resistance is normal. It is often emotional, not logical. Leaders must recognise resistance as communication, not defiance.

8.4.1 Identifying the Reasons for Resistance

Common reasons include:

- Fear of loss (status, competence, security)
- Uncertainty about the future
- Lack of trust in leadership
- Workload pressure
- Poor communication
- Previous negative experiences of change
- Perceived unfairness
- Feeling excluded from decisions

Understanding the reason allows leaders to respond constructively.

8.4.2 Tools for Addressing Concerns

Leaders should:

- Invite honest feedback
- Use one-to-one and team discussions
- Address practical and emotional concerns
- Provide reassurance grounded in facts
- Clarify expectations and timelines
- Adjust plans where appropriate
- Demonstrate empathy and patience

Staff rarely resist change itself they resist *how* change is implemented.

8.4.3 Reinforcement and Sustainability

To embed change:

- Celebrate early successes
- Monitor progress regularly
- Provide refresher training
- Align performance expectations
- Update policies and procedures
- Share positive feedback from patients and staff
- Maintain visible leadership support

Sustainability is achieved when new behaviours become the norm not the exception.

8.5 Measuring and Evaluating Change Outcomes

Change must produce measurable improvements. Leaders must evaluate:

8.5.1 Key Performance Indicators (KPIs)

These may relate to:

- Patient outcomes
- Staff satisfaction
- Safety incidents
- Waiting times
- Budget performance
- Clinical audit results
- Workflow efficiency

KPIs must be relevant, realistic, and regularly monitored.

8.5.2 Feedback Mechanisms and Continuous Improvement

Effective mechanisms include:

- Patient and family feedback
- Staff surveys and focus groups
- Learning from incidents
- After-action reviews
- Regular progress reports
- Quality improvement dashboards

Continuous improvement ensures that change is not a one-off event but an ongoing commitment.

Conclusion

Leading change in healthcare requires a blend of strategic thinking, emotional intelligence, communication skill, and operational discipline. It requires leaders to understand human behaviour, manage uncertainty, build trust, and maintain momentum in the face of pressures and resistance.

Successful change is never about imposing directives—it is about guiding people through transition, supporting their development, and embedding new ways of working that improve safety, quality, and patient experience.

Leaders who master the art of change become catalysts for transformation in systems that desperately need innovation and resilience. In the UK and Ireland, where reform agendas are ambitious and workforce pressures intense, effective change leadership is not optional it is essential.

CHAPTER 9

Conflict Resolution and Negotiation

Conflict is an unavoidable part of healthcare. High workloads, emotional stress, multidisciplinary teams, limited resources, and differing clinical perspectives all contribute to tension. How leaders respond to conflict determines whether it becomes destructive or whether it becomes a catalyst for learning, improvement, and stronger relationships.

Negotiation is equally essential. Healthcare leaders frequently negotiate resources, staff allocations, rota changes, interdepartmental agreements, patient pathways, and partnership arrangements across diverse organisations.

This chapter provides leaders with practical tools, emotional intelligence strategies, and structured approaches to managing conflict and negotiating effectively within the complex environments of the NHS, HSE, and wider health systems.

9.1 Nature and Sources of Conflict in Healthcare Settings

Conflict arises when expectations, values, needs, or perceptions differ. In healthcare, these differences often occur under intense pressure, making conflict more likely and more emotionally charged.

9.1.1 Interpersonal Conflict

Examples include:

- Personality clashes
- Miscommunication
- Perceived unfairness
- Differences in working styles
- Emotionally charged interactions after stressful shifts

Leaders must address interpersonal conflict early to prevent escalation.

9.1.2 Intergroup and Interdepartmental Conflict

Healthcare relies on collaboration between:

- Departments
- Clinical specialties
- Multidisciplinary teams
- Administrative and clinical functions

Common sources include:

- Competing priorities (e.g. bed management vs elective surgery)
- Role ambiguity
- Lack of clarity about responsibilities
- Poor communication pathways
- Resource scarcity
- Differences in departmental culture

These conflicts affect patient flow, morale, and service quality.

9.1.3 Organisational Conflict

Examples:

- Resistance to change
- Disputes about new policies
- Rota redesign
- Workload distribution
- Complaints about leadership decisions

Leaders must balance empathy with clarity about organisational needs.

9.1.4 Clinical or Ethical Conflict

These conflicts arise from:

- Differences in clinical judgement
- Disagreements about treatment decisions
- Patient safety concerns
- Moral distress among staff

Leaders must ensure open discussion, clear escalation pathways, and a supportive learning culture.

9.2 Conflict Resolution Strategies for Healthcare Leaders

Effective conflict resolution requires emotional intelligence, structure, and a non-defensive approach. Leaders must remain objective, fair, and solutions-focused.

9.2.1 Interest-Based Approach

This approach separates the *people* from the *problem*.

Steps:

1. Identify underlying interests (not just stated positions)

2. Explore each party's concerns, needs, and motivations

3. Seek options that address shared interests

4. Agree a solution that benefits the team and organisation

Example:
Two clinicians dispute over theatre access. The real issue is not the schedule it is workload imbalance and communication gaps. Resolving the underlying issues creates long-term improvement.

9.2.2 Mediation Techniques

Leaders act as neutral facilitators.

Effective mediation involves:

- Setting ground rules for respectful discussion
- Allowing each party to speak uninterrupted
- Summarising perspectives neutrally
- Identifying shared goals (e.g. patient safety)
- Encouraging collaborative problem-solving
- Clarifying next steps and accountability

Mediation reduces defensiveness and restores trust.

9.2.3 Effective Communication in Conflict Resolution

Leaders should use:

- Open-ended questions
- Reflective listening ("What I hear you saying is...")
- Neutral language
- Calm tone
- A focus on behaviours, not personal attributes
- Clear summarisation of agreements

Emotionally intelligent communication helps de-escalate tension.

9.3 Negotiation Skills in Healthcare Leadership

Negotiation is a core leadership skill. Healthcare leaders negotiate daily often without realising it.

9.3.1 Principles of Effective Negotiation

Key principles include:

1. Preparation

Understand your goals, the other party's goals, constraints, and desired outcomes.

2. Clear Communication

Present proposals concisely and confidently.

3. Collaboration Over Competition

Seek mutual benefit, not "winners" and "losers."

4. Flexibility

Identify areas of compromise and areas that are non-negotiable.

5. Emotional Intelligence

Stay calm, professional, and respectful even when the other party is under strain.

6. Closing with Clarity

Confirm decisions, responsibilities, and timelines in writing if necessary.

9.3.2 Types of Negotiation in Healthcare

Intra-organisational Negotiation

- Staffing levels
- Budget priorities
- Clinical rota management
- Equipment procurement
- Interdepartmental collaboration

Inter-organisational Negotiation

- Pathway redesign across ICSs
- Partnerships within Sláintecare Community Networks
- Agreements with voluntary or private providers
- Joint initiatives with local authorities

Negotiating with External Stakeholders

- Regulators
- Unions
- Academic institutions
- Community groups
- Patient advocates

Healthcare leaders must balance assertiveness with diplomacy.

9.3.3 Ethical Considerations in Negotiation

Leaders must remain:

- Transparent
- Fair
- Accountable
- Respectful of boundaries
- Focused on patient safety and staff wellbeing

Ethical negotiation builds long-term trust and credibility.

9.4 Building and Maintaining Professional Relationships in the UK and Ireland Health Systems

Relationships are the currency of effective leadership. Leaders who invest in relationships create resilient, high-performing teams.

9.4.1 Relationship Building With Peers and Teams

Strong relationships require:

- Approachability
- Integrity
- Reliability
- Genuine interest in others
- Visible support during difficult periods
- Celebrating achievements
- Respect across all professional roles

Leaders who are consistent and fair develop staff commitment and loyalty.

9.4.2 Collaboration Across Multidisciplinary Teams

Collaboration is central to safe patient care.

Leaders should:

• Encourage cross-disciplinary respect
• Facilitate shared decision-making
• Promote structured communication tools (SBAR, huddles, MDT meetings)
• Address conflict promptly
• Support relational resilience

In both the NHS and HSE, integrated care requires leaders to bridge traditional boundaries.

9.4.3 Managing External Relationships

Externally, leaders must maintain strong relationships with:

• Voluntary and community partners
• Mental health and social care providers
• Regulators and inspectors
• Commissioners / CHOs / ICBs
• Universities and training bodies
• Public representatives and the media

Professionalism, transparency, and preparedness are essential.

Conclusion

Conflict and negotiation are unavoidable in healthcare but they are also opportunities for growth, improvement, and strengthened relationships. Leaders who understand the causes of conflict, respond with emotional intelligence, and negotiate with integrity create environments where staff trust one another, communication is open, and patient care remains the central focus.

In the complex systems of the UK and Ireland, leaders who excel at conflict resolution and negotiation will be better positioned to navigate competing demands, influence across organisational boundaries, and build collaborative cultures essential for safe and effective healthcare.

CHAPTER 10

Quality and Performance Improvement

High-quality care is the foundation of every healthcare system. Patients expect and deserve safe, effective, compassionate, person-centred services. Regulators demand transparent accountability.

Staff need clear processes, support, and a culture that enables them to deliver their best work. Organisations must balance quality with efficiency, resource pressures, and growing demand.

This chapter explores the core components of quality improvement (QI) and performance management in healthcare. It provides practical tools, frameworks, and insights that leaders can apply to drive sustainable improvements in the NHS, HSE, voluntary hospitals, and community health services.

10.1 Importance of Quality in Healthcare

Quality is not an abstract concept; it directly affects patient outcomes, staff satisfaction, organisational reputation, and the public's trust.

Across the UK and Ireland, quality in healthcare is defined using similar dimensions.

10.1.1 Definitions and Dimensions of Quality

UK: CQC's Five Key Lines of Enquiry (KLOEs)

Services must be:

1. **Safe**

2. **Effective**

3. **Caring**

4. **Responsive**

5. **Well-led**

Ireland: HIQA's Six Dimensions of Quality

1. **Safe care**

2. **Timely access**

3. **Effective services**

4. **Person-centred care**

5. **Efficient use of resources**

6. **Staff and leadership involvement**

These frameworks guide inspection, regulation, improvement, and performance assessment.

10.1.2 The Role of Leaders in Quality Improvement (QI)

Quality improvement is a leadership responsibility not just a clinical or operational task.

Leaders must:

• Set the tone for safety and learning
• Encourage staff to speak up
• Support data-driven decision-making
• Ensure robust systems for audit, monitoring, and evaluation
• Communicate transparently

• Foster a culture of continuous improvement and psychological safety

When leaders model curiosity, accountability, and openness, quality naturally strengthens.

10.2 Performance Measures and Indicators in the UK and Ireland Healthcare Systems

What gets measured gets improved. Performance indicators provide a structured way to assess whether services are meeting expectations.

10.2.1 Key Performance Indicators (KPIs)

KPIs measure:

• Safety
• Quality
• Efficiency
• Patient outcomes
• Workforce wellbeing
• Financial performance
• Access and timeliness

Examples include:

• Waiting times (A&E, outpatients, diagnostics)
• Hospital-acquired infection rates
• Medication error rates
• Staff turnover and absenteeism

• Patient experience scores (Friends & Family Test,
National Patient Survey)

• Length of stay metrics

• Compliance with clinical guidelines

• Response times for community and mental health
services

KPIs must be meaningful, measurable, and aligned with
strategic goals.

10.2.2 Balanced Scorecard for Healthcare Leaders

A balanced scorecard examines performance across
four domains:

1. **Patient/Service User Perspective**

    o Safety, satisfaction, outcomes

2. **Internal Processes**

    o Efficiency, compliance, incident trends

3. **Learning and Growth**

    o Staff training, wellbeing, innovation

4. **Financial Sustainability**

    o Budget performance, cost-saving
       initiatives

This holistic approach ensures leaders do not focus
solely on one dimension at the expense of others.

10.2.3 Use of Data and Analytic Tools in Performance Monitoring

Data is essential for modern healthcare improvement.

Leaders should use:

- Dashboards
- Statistical Process Control (SPC) charts
- Audit reports
- Benchmarking
- Quality metrics from EHR systems
- Incident and complaints analytics
- Workforce data (turnover, sickness, skill mix)

Data helps leaders identify trends, highlight risks, and evaluate the effectiveness of improvement actions.

10.3 Quality Improvement Methodologies in Healthcare

Quality improvement is a structured discipline grounded in evidence-based tools and methodologies.

10.3.1 Plan-Do-Study-Act (PDSA)

A widely used method in both the NHS and HSE.

PLAN

Define the problem, gather baseline data, and design interventions.

DO

Test the intervention on a small scale.

STUDY

Analyse the results what worked and what did not?

ACT

Adjust and scale up if successful OR refine and test again.

PDSA promotes iterative learning rather than large-scale, high-risk implementation.

10.3.2 Lean Principles

Lean focuses on eliminating waste and improving flow. Waste includes:

- Waiting
- Overproduction
- Errors/rework
- Unnecessary movement
- Poor communication
- Underutilised staff skills

Lean thinking encourages staff to identify inefficiencies and create smoother processes that improve patient experiences.

10.3.3 Six Sigma in Healthcare

Six Sigma reduces variation and defects in processes. Tools include:

- DMAIC (Define, Measure, Analyse, Improve, Control)
- Root cause analysis
- Statistical analysis
- Process mapping

Though more technical, it is useful for major clinical and operational improvements.

10.3.4 Root Cause Analysis (RCA)

Used for significant incidents or near-misses.

Steps include:

1. Data gathering

2. Chronology creation

3. Identification of contributory factors

4. Categorisation (human factors, system failures, environment, communication)

5. Development of actionable recommendations

The goal is learning not blame.

10.4 Clinical Governance and Patient Safety

Clinical governance provides a framework for continuous improvement in patient care.

10.4.1 Clinical Audit

Audit compares practice against standards.

Examples:

- Compliance with infection control policies
- Medication prescribing accuracy
- Surgical checklist adherence
- Falls assessment documentation

Audit cycles must include re-audit to ensure improvements are sustained.

10.4.2 Risk Management

Healthcare is inherently risky.

Risk management includes:

- Incident reporting
- Risk registers
- Trend analysis
- Early warning systems
- Staff training
- Simulation exercises
- Lessons-learned reviews

Both HIQA and CQC expect clear evidence of risk management processes.

10.4.3 Safety Culture and Just Culture

A just culture balances accountability with learning.

Characteristics include:

• Encouraging staff to speak up
• Avoiding blame for honest mistakes
• Holding individuals accountable for reckless behaviour
• Learning from incidents systemically
• Supporting staff involved in incidents (second victim support)

Leaders set the tone for safety culture through their responses to errors.

10.5 Continuous Improvement and Innovation

Great organisations do not wait for problems they continuously aim to improve.

10.5.1 Fostering an Innovative Culture

Innovation thrives when staff feel:

- Safe to share ideas
- Supported to test solutions
- Respected for their expertise
- Empowered to challenge outdated practices

Leaders must remove fear and create space for improvement.

10.5.2 Learning from Outcomes and Feedback

Improvement sources include:

- Patient feedback
- Staff surveys
- Complaints and compliments
- Incident review outcomes
- Audit results
- Benchmarking across organisations
- Longitudinal performance data

Learning organisations ask: "What does this teach us?" rather than "Who is at fault?"

10.5.3 Leadership's Role in Driving Quality Improvement

Leaders must:

- Allocate time and resources for QI
- Provide training and capacity-building
- Celebrate successes
- Remove barriers to improvement
- Encourage multidisciplinary involvement
- Model curiosity and continuous learning

When leaders consistently prioritise quality, it becomes embedded in the organisation's identity.

Conclusion

Quality and performance improvement are continuous, not occasional tasks. They must be woven into the daily practice of every healthcare professional. Strong leadership, a supportive culture, evidence-based methodologies, and reliable data systems drive sustainable improvement.

Healthcare organisations in the UK and Ireland face growing pressures but with the right tools, culture, and leadership behaviours, they can deliver safer, more effective, more compassionate care while maintaining organisational stability and public trust.

CHAPTER 11

Cross-Cultural Understanding and Professionalism

Healthcare in the UK and Ireland is delivered within highly diverse societies. Patients, families, and staff come from a wide range of cultural, ethnic, linguistic, religious, and social backgrounds. Effective care therefore requires more than clinical expertise it requires cultural awareness, humility, and professionalism. Leaders must model behaviours that create inclusive environments where all individuals are respected, valued, and treated equitably.

This chapter explores the importance of cultural competence, the challenges and opportunities created by diversity, and the professional standards that underpin safe and respectful practice.

11.1 Cultural Competence and Sensitivity in Healthcare

Cultural competence is the ability to understand, appreciate, and interact effectively with people from different cultural backgrounds. It is essential for delivering safe, person-centred care.

11.1.1 Understanding Cultural Diversity

The UK and Ireland both have increasingly multicultural populations, shaped by:

- Economic migration
- Asylum and refugee movements
- International healthcare workers
- Travelling communities
- Varied religious identities
- Generational cultural shifts

These populations bring different:

- Health beliefs
- Communication styles
- Expectations of care
- Attitudes toward medication, treatment, and mental health
- Traditions and customs
- Family dynamics and decision-making processes

Healthcare leaders must ensure staff are equipped to recognise and respond appropriately to these differences.

11.1.2 Overcoming Cultural Barriers

Barriers to effective care may include:

- Language differences
- Low health literacy
- Distrust of healthcare systems
- Stigma around certain illnesses
- Different beliefs about pain, treatment, or death

- Gender or family role expectations
- Cultural experiences of authority

Leaders must ensure:

- Access to professional interpreters
- Culturally sensitive communication materials
- Clear consent processes
- Respect for cultural and religious practices
- Staff training to reduce unconscious bias
- Collaboration with community groups

Inclusive care improves outcomes, satisfaction, and engagement.

11.1.3 Effective Communication Across Cultures

Culturally competent communication involves:

- Avoiding jargon
- Speaking plainly and respectfully
- Checking for understanding
- Using interpreters rather than family members
- Being aware of non-verbal communication differences
- Showing patience and empathy
- Recognising cultural norms regarding eye contact, touch, or decision-making

Good communication builds trust and ensures informed, safe care.

11.2 Ethical and Professional Behaviour in Healthcare

Professionalism is the foundation of trust between healthcare providers and the communities they serve. It requires integrity, responsibility, accountability, and respect.

11.2.1 Ethical Principles

Healthcare ethics is grounded in four core principles:

1. Autonomy

Respecting individuals' rights to make informed decisions.

2. Beneficence

Acting in the best interests of the patient.

3. Non-Maleficence

Avoiding harm.

4. Justice

Ensuring fairness and equity in access and treatment.

Leaders reinforce these principles by modelling ethical practice and ensuring staff receive guidance and training on ethical decision-making.

11.2.2 Confidentiality and Data Protection

Confidentiality is essential for maintaining trust.

Leaders must ensure:

• Compliance with GDPR and data protection
legislation
• Secure handling of records
• Training on confidentiality policies
• Appropriate sharing of information on a need-to-know
basis
• Clear governance around digital systems and access
rights

Breach of confidentiality damages trust and can have
serious legal consequences.

11.2.3 Professional Boundaries

Professional boundaries protect both patients and
staff.

Leaders must ensure that boundaries are maintained in
relation to:

• Dual relationships
• Communication with patients (including social media)
• Emotional boundaries and over-involvement
• Gift-giving or receiving
• Confidentiality beyond the clinical setting

Clear boundaries safeguard professionalism and protect organisational reputation.

11.3 Importance of Cultural Sensitivity in Patient Care

Culturally sensitive care improves outcomes, reduces risk, and strengthens relationships with patients and families.

11.3.1 Patient-Centred Approaches

Cultural sensitivity aligns with person-centred care, where each patient is seen as an individual.

This includes:

• Understanding their cultural background
• Respecting beliefs, preferences, and values
• Involving families where appropriate
• Adapting care plans based on cultural needs
• Offering privacy and dignity
• Ensuring equitable access

Patient-centred care is a regulatory expectation under both CQC and HIQA standards.

11.3.2 Stereotyping and Bias in Healthcare

Bias can be conscious or unconscious. If unaddressed, it can influence clinical decisions, communication quality, and patient engagement.

Examples include bias based on:

- Ethnicity
- Age
- Gender
- Social class
- Disability
- Traveller or Roma identity
- Mental health history
- Addiction or substance use

Leaders must actively challenge stereotypes, encourage reflection, and promote a culture of equality and respect.

11.3.3 Strategies for Providing Inclusive Care

Leaders should support staff by ensuring:

- Access to cultural awareness training
- Policies that respect religious and cultural practices (dietary needs, dress, modesty, end-of-life rituals)
- Clear processes for interpreter services
- Inclusive signage and communication materials
- Culturally safe environments

• Collaboration with cultural mediators and community organisations

This strengthens trust and improves care for all groups.

11.4 Developing Cross-Cultural Competencies

Cultural competence is not static; it is built over time through education, experience, reflection, and engagement.

11.4.1 Continuous Learning and Education

Effective training includes:

• Cultural awareness programmes
• Equality, diversity, and inclusion (EDI) modules
• Unconscious bias training
• Workshops with community partners
• Case-based scenarios and reflective practice exercises
• Training aligned with HIQA, CQC, NHS, and HSE frameworks

Leaders must champion and prioritise such training.

11.4.2 Reflective Practice

Reflection allows staff to:

- Explore their own cultural assumptions
- Understand emotional responses
- Learn from challenging interactions
- Recognise bias
- Improve communication strategies

Reflection is central to professional regulation across nursing, medicine, and allied health.

11.4.3 Building a Culturally Competent Healthcare Workforce

Leaders can strengthen the workforce by:

- Recruiting diverse staff
- Supporting international healthcare workers
- Encouraging multilingual staff to assist appropriately
- Creating peer support networks
- Providing structured induction for new cultural contexts
- Ensuring equity in promotion and leadership opportunities

Diversity enriches organisational culture and improves care quality.

Conclusion

Cross-cultural understanding and professionalism are essential competencies for every healthcare leader. In diverse societies like the UK and Ireland, culturally sensitive care is not optional—it is fundamental to safety, dignity, and equity.

Leaders who embody professional values, challenge bias, respect cultural differences, and promote inclusive practices help create environments where both staff and patients feel respected and understood. This strengthens relationships, enhances patient experience, improves outcomes, and aligns with regulatory expectations for safe, compassionate, well-led services.

CHAPTER 12

Leadership in Action: Case Studies and Practical Applications

Healthcare leadership is most clearly demonstrated not in theory, but in action. Leaders must navigate complexity, manage uncertainty, coordinate multidisciplinary teams, and make decisions that influence safety, staff morale, and patient outcomes.

This chapter presents practical case studies that illustrate how leadership principles apply in real scenarios across acute, community, and primary care settings.

Each case study highlights critical challenges, examines leadership responses, and outlines lessons applicable to the UK and Ireland's healthcare environments.

12.1 Case Studies Illustrating Leadership in Healthcare

The following case studies reflect common challenges: high-pressure environments, workforce crises, communication failures, ethical dilemmas, and system-wide constraints.

They are designed to show how leaders can apply emotional intelligence, strategic thinking, compassion, and evidence-based decision-making.

Case Study 1: Managing a Multidisciplinary Team in a Busy Hospital Ward

Background

A large acute hospital ward experiences high staff turnover, increasing agency spend, multiple clinical incidents, and declining patient experience scores.

Nursing staff report feeling overwhelmed and unsupported. Medical staff raise concerns about communication breakdowns and delayed decision-making.

The ward is rated "Requires Improvement" for safety and leadership in a recent internal audit.

Leadership Challenges

• Fragmented communication between nursing, medical, and allied health professionals
• Low morale and fatigue among staff
• Inefficient ward rounds causing delays in care
• Confusion around roles and accountability
• Lack of psychological safety staff reluctant to raise concerns
• High sickness absence impacting staffing stability

Leadership Response

The ward leader introduces a structured improvement plan:

1. Rebuilding psychological safety

• Conducts listening sessions with staff
• Establishes a "no-blame" philosophy
• Encourages reporting of near-misses and ideas

2. Improving communication

- Introduces structured MDT huddles three times daily
- Uses SBAR for consistent communication
- Implements a shared digital task list

3. Clarifying roles

- Revises role descriptions
- Delegates appropriately based on skills and experience
- Encourages autonomy for senior nurses and team leads

4. Supporting staff wellbeing

- Ensures protected breaks
- Introduces peer-support circles
- Sets up wellbeing sessions after difficult events

5. Continuous improvement

- Uses PDSA cycles to redesign ward rounds
- Monitors KPIs such as delays, patient experience, and safety metrics
- Shares short-term wins to motivate the team

Outcomes

- Improved teamwork and morale
- Reduction in medication errors
- Better patient flow and shorter length of stay
- Positive staff feedback
- Improved compliance with quality standards

Key Lessons

• Leadership visibility and psychological safety are essential
• Small, consistent changes can transform performance
• Clear communication structures improve safety and efficiency
• Staff engagement drives sustainable improvement

Case Study 2: Coordinating Care for a Patient with Complex Needs

Background

A patient with multiple long-term conditions diabetes, COPD, depression, and limited mobility experiences repeated hospital admissions. Communication between primary care, mental health services, community teams, and family is poor. The patient feels unsupported and frustrated.

Leadership Challenges

• Fragmented services and unclear ownership
• Poor information sharing
• Differing priorities across agencies
• Family feeling excluded from decision-making
• Social determinants contributing to poor outcomes

Leadership Response

A community team leader creates a coordinated, person-centred care plan:

1. Establishing a case conference

• Brings GP, consultant, mental health nurse, social worker, community physiotherapist, and family together
• Identifies shared goals and responsibilities

2. Developing a holistic plan

• Addresses medical, psychological, and social needs
• Includes family involvement where appropriate
• Uses a single shared care document

3. Enhancing communication

• Creates a central digital record accessible to all services
• Assigns a named care coordinator

4. Monitoring progress

• Holds review meetings every six weeks
• Tracks admissions, medication adherence, and wellbeing

Outcomes

• Reduction in hospital admissions
• Improved medication management
• Stronger patient engagement with mental health

supports
• Family satisfaction improves significantly

Key Lessons

• Coordinated care prevents crisis and improves
outcomes
• Shared goals bridge organisational boundaries
• Patient and family engagement must be intentional
• Leaders must advocate for whole-system
collaboration

Case Study 3: Handling Operational Challenges During a Crisis

Background

A winter surge results in full emergency departments,
delayed discharges, staff shortages, and rising tension
among teams. Junior staff feel unsupported, while
senior leaders feel pressure to meet national targets.

Leadership Challenges

• Overcrowding and safety risks
• Workforce fatigue
• Competing priorities: flow versus safety
• Limited resources
• High emotional pressure

Leadership Response

A senior operational lead implements crisis management strategies:

1. Activation of a clear escalation framework

• Opens surge capacity areas
• Mobilises additional staffing from non-clinical areas
• Prioritises high-risk patients

2. Improved communication

• Sets up hourly huddles between ED, bed management, and wards
• Provides honest updates to staff

3. Protecting staff morale

• Rotates breaks to reduce burnout
• Facilitates rapid debriefing sessions after critical events

4. Working with external partners

• Engages community services to accelerate safe discharges
• Collaborates with social care and private providers

5. Focus on learning

• Conducts post-crisis reviews
• Identifies what worked well and areas for improvement

Outcomes

- Reduced waiting times
- Safer patient flow
- Improved staff cohesion
- Stronger resilience for future surges

Key Lessons

- Calm, structured leadership is essential during crisis
- Real-time communication prevents chaos
- Supporting staff emotionally is part of operational leadership
- Cross-system collaboration accelerates solutions

Conclusion

These case studies demonstrate that healthcare leadership is not merely about holding authority—it is about influencing behaviour, shaping culture, and guiding teams through complexity with clarity and compassion.

Effective leaders:

- Listen deeply
- Communicate clearly
- Act decisively
- Support staff wellbeing
- Build trust across disciplines
- Use evidence and data to guide decisions

- Seek collaboration rather than control
- Learn from every challenge

Leadership in action is visible in the smallest interactions and the largest system decisions. It is the thread that holds safe, high-performing healthcare together.

CHAPTER 13

Future Directions in Healthcare Leadership

Healthcare is undergoing one of the most significant periods of transformation in modern history. Demographic pressures, workforce shortages, technological advances, shifting public expectations, widening health inequalities, and new models of integrated care are reshaping systems in both the UK and Ireland. Future healthcare leaders must be agile, informed, compassionate, and strategically focused if they are to navigate these evolving challenges successfully.

This chapter explores the major trends influencing the future of healthcare leadership and outlines the capabilities leaders must develop to thrive in a dynamic, complex, and often unpredictable environment.

13.1 Trends Shaping the Future of Healthcare in the UK and Ireland

Several macro-level trends are redefining health systems and placing new demands on leaders.

13.1.1 Technological Advancements and Digital Transformation

Technology is transforming healthcare delivery.

Key trends include:

• Artificial intelligence (AI) for diagnostics, risk prediction, scheduling, triage, and workflow optimisation
• Robotics in surgery, rehabilitation, and logistics
• Telehealth and virtual care for chronic disease management
• Electronic health records becoming more integrated and interoperable
• Wearable technology and remote monitoring
• Automated medication dispensing and digital prescribing
• Big data analytics for population health management

Leaders must ensure technology adoption is safe, user-friendly, evidence-based, and aligned with service needs not simply pursued for its novelty.

13.1.2 Growing Diversity in the Healthcare Workforce

The health workforce is increasingly multicultural.

Future leaders must:

• Support international recruits
• Promote inclusive cultures
• Ensure equitable career development
• Address bias and discrimination proactively
• Provide cultural competence training
• Build psychologically safe environments for diverse staff

Diversity is a strategic strength that improves innovation, insight, and patient experience.

13.1.3 Rising Patient and Public Expectations

Patients expect:

• Faster access
• Greater transparency
• More involvement in decisions
• Better communication
• Consistency and continuity
• Compassion and dignity
• Culturally sensitive care

This shift requires leaders to excel in service design, patient engagement, and experience-led improvement.

13.1.4 Increasing Emphasis on Interdisciplinary Collaboration

Integrated care systems (ICSs), CHOs, community networks, and cross-agency partnerships will continue to grow.

Leaders must work across:

- Primary and secondary care
- Community and voluntary sectors
- Mental health and social care
- Education, housing, and justice partners
- Independent and private providers

The future leader must be a system leader not just an organisational leader.

13.2 Preparing Future Leaders for the Evolving Healthcare Landscape

Emerging leaders need a new skillset that extends beyond traditional management.

13.2.1 Leadership Development Programmes

Leadership pipelines must include:

- Emerging leader programmes
- Talent management pathways
- Executive mentorship

- Coaching and reflective practice
- Cross-sector placements
- Exposure to multidisciplinary leadership
- Training aligned with CQC, HIQA, NHS, and HSE expectations

Investing in leadership is investing in organisational resilience.

13.2.2 Enhancing Emotional Intelligence in Leaders

Future leaders must excel in:

- Self-awareness
- Empathy
- Emotional regulation
- Conflict resolution
- Authentic communication
- Relational trust-building

Emotional intelligence will be as valuable as technical competence.

13.2.3 Adapting to New Leadership Theories and Practices

The next decade will see increased emphasis on:

- Compassionate leadership
- Distributed leadership
- Inclusive leadership

- Trauma-informed leadership
- Systems leadership
- Strengths-based approaches

These models reinforce collaboration, wellbeing, and shared responsibility.

13.3 Challenges and Opportunities in Future Healthcare Leadership

Future leaders must be ready to address challenges with creativity, confidence, and strategic foresight.

13.3.1 Navigating Complex Healthcare Systems

Challenges include:

- Fragmentation
- Bureaucracy
- Political influence
- Workforce shortages
- Increasing demand
- Budget constraints

Effective leaders will:

- Influence across boundaries
- Build strong stakeholder relationships
- Align teams around shared goals
- Simplify complexity where possible
- Advocate for sustainable, patient-centred solutions

13.3.2 Balancing Operational Demands and Strategic Objectives

Daily pressures can overwhelm leaders.

The most successful future leaders will:

- Protect strategic thinking time
- Delegate effectively
- Build strong operational teams
- Use data to make informed decisions
- Avoid reactive, crisis-driven management
- Focus on long-term outcomes

Balancing the urgent with the important is essential.

13.3.3 Leading Through Uncertainty

Healthcare is facing:

- Rapid technological change
- Evolving disease patterns
- Climate-related health pressures
- Policy fluctuation
- Workforce volatility

Leaders must cultivate:

- Resilience
- Adaptability
- Critical thinking

- Scenario planning
- Calm, steady communication

Uncertainty is now the normal operating environment.

Conclusion

The future of healthcare leadership will demand more of leaders than ever before. They must combine strategic insight with compassion, emotional intelligence with analytical skill, and stability with adaptability. They must create cultures where staff feel valued and supported, where patients feel heard and respected, and where improvement is continuous and embedded.

Healthcare in the UK and Ireland will continue to evolve rapidly. Leaders who embrace change, invest in their development, empower their teams, and maintain unwavering commitment to quality and safety will shape the future of healthcare for the better.

The next generation of leaders will not simply manage services they will transform them.

CONCLUSION

Healthcare leadership in the UK and Ireland is undergoing a profound transformation.

The environments in which leaders operate are becoming increasingly complex, fast-moving, and emotionally demanding. The pressures of rising patient expectations, regulatory scrutiny, financial challenges, workforce shortages, technological shifts, and wider social inequalities require leaders who can think systemically, act ethically, communicate authentically, and inspire confidence even in times of uncertainty.

Throughout this book, we have explored the essential domains of modern healthcare leadership: understanding systems and structures; building multidisciplinary relationships; managing people, resources, and performance; navigating conflict and negotiation; leading change; embedding quality and safety; and engaging with cultural competence, professionalism, and inclusive practice. These are not theoretical concepts they are daily realities for anyone entrusted with leading teams and services in healthcare.

A consistent theme has emerged across every chapter: leadership is fundamentally relational. It is about people not processes, metrics, or organisational charts. The most influential leaders are those who create cultures of trust, psychological safety, curiosity, respect, and continuous improvement. They listen deeply, communicate clearly, and foster environments where staff feel valued, empowered, and supported to deliver their best work.

They combine compassionate behaviour with accountability, ensuring high standards of care while recognising the pressures and humanity of the workforce.

Equally important is a leader's commitment to learning. Healthcare will continue to evolve, shaped by demographic changes, policy reform, technological innovation, and global health challenges. Leaders who remain open to new thinking, reflective in their practice, willing to question assumptions, and proactive about their development will be best placed to guide their organisations through whatever the future holds.

Finally, leadership is an act of service. Leaders exist to support staff, champion patients, uphold public trust, and ensure that care is safe, equitable, and compassionate. The responsibility is significant but so too is the opportunity for impact. Strong, values-driven leadership has the power to transform teams, enhance patient outcomes, strengthen system performance, and improve the lives of communities across the UK and Ireland.

As the healthcare landscape continues to shift, this book provides a foundation for current and aspiring leaders to reflect, develop, and refine their practice. The next generation of leaders will not simply manage the system they will shape it.

This is the work of leadership. This is the work of change. And this is the work that defines the future of healthcare.

APPENDICES

APPENDIX A: LEADERSHIP REFLECTION TOOLS

Reflection is an essential part of effective leadership. It enables leaders to evaluate decisions, understand behaviours, recognise emotional triggers, and refine their practice.

Below are three structured tools you can use for leadership development, supervision, or appraisal processes.

A1. The Leadership Reflection Cycle

A simple but powerful model encouraging structured reflection after events, decisions, or challenging interactions.

1. What happened?

- **Describe the event objectively.**
- **What decisions were made?**
- **Who was involved?**

2. What did I think and feel?

• What emotions did this situation bring up?
• Were these emotions helpful or unhelpful?

3. What went well?

• What actions were effective?
• What leadership behaviours strengthened performance?

4. What could have gone better?

• What barriers or limitations appeared?
• What would you change next time?

5. What will I do differently now?

• Identify one concrete action you will implement.
• How will this improve future leadership practice?

A2. The 360° Leadership Reflection Template

Designed to support structured feedback from colleagues, managers, and direct reports.

Domains for Reflection

1. Communication

   o   Do I communicate clearly?

   o   Do staff understand expectations?

2. Decision-Making

- o   Are my decisions timely and evidence-based?

3. Emotional Intelligence

- o   Do I manage stress effectively?

- o   Do I respond constructively to conflict?

4. Team Support & Development

- o   Do I empower staff?

- o   Do I recognise achievements regularly?

5. Values & Professionalism

- o   Do my actions reflect organisational values?

- o   Do I maintain fairness and integrity?

Rating Scale (1–5)

1 = rarely demonstrated
5 = consistently demonstrated

Include space for free-text comments to deepen the feedback.

A3. Reflective Practice Questions for Healthcare Leaders

These prompts are designed for journal writing, coaching, or annual leadership reviews.

Self-Awareness

- What leadership behaviour of mine had the biggest impact this month?
- When did I feel most challenged, and why?
- What assumptions did I make today, and were they accurate?

Team Leadership

- How did I contribute to team morale this week?
- What feedback am I avoiding giving?
- How did I create psychological safety today?

Systems Thinking

- What system pressures influenced my decisions?
- Did I consider the wider organisation when making choices?

Professional Values

- How did I model compassion, clarity, or accountability today?
- What behaviour of mine did not align with my leadership values?

These questions help leaders evaluate their actions in a structured, meaningful way.

APPENDIX B: LEADERSHIP COMPETENCY FRAMEWORKS

Below is a concise, practical competency framework tailored to healthcare leadership in the UK and Ireland. It can be used for recruitment, appraisal, supervision, and personal development planning.

B1. Core Leadership Competencies

1. Strategic Thinking

- Understand broader system priorities
- Align team objectives to organisational goals
- Interpret data and evidence to guide planning
- Anticipate challenges and create contingency plans

2. People Leadership

- Build trust and motivate diverse teams
- Provide constructive feedback
- Address performance issues fairly
- Promote wellbeing and psychological safety
- Resolve conflict confidently

3. Communication Excellence

- Communicate clearly, consistently, and respectfully
- Adapt style to audience and context

• Demonstrate active listening and emotional intelligence
• Facilitate collaborative discussion

4. Professionalism and Integrity

• Model ethical decision-making
• Maintain confidentiality and boundaries
• Demonstrate fairness, respect, and cultural competence
• Uphold organisational values

5. Quality and Safety Focus

• Monitor KPIs and performance data
• Lead improvement initiatives
• Understand regulatory standards (CQC, HIQA, MHC)
• Promote a just culture and learning from incidents

6. Change Leadership

• Apply structured change models (e.g., Lewin, Kotter)
• Engage staff and stakeholders
• Communicate clearly during transition
• Sustain improvements through reinforcement

7. Systems Leadership

• Work across organisational boundaries
• Understand primary, secondary, community, and voluntary sector interdependencies

- Promote integration and shared problem-solving
- Support population health priorities

B2. Leadership Competency Self-Assessment Tool

Leaders rate each competency from 1–5:

1 = limited ability
3 = developing
5 = highly proficient

Below each domain, leaders list:

- Evidence of competency
- Areas for development
- Suggested training or support

This tool forms a foundation for annual personal development plans.

B3. Mapping Competencies to Organisational Role Levels

Entry/Emerging Leaders

- Strong communication
- Self-awareness
- Learning mindset
- Support team coordination

Mid-Level Leaders

• Performance management
• Service planning
• Managing complex teams
• Leading quality improvement projects

Senior Leaders/Executives

• System leadership
• Strategic design and policy interpretation
• Organisational culture shaping
• Governance and accountability frameworks

This ensures development is tailored to level and responsibility.

APPENDIX C: LEADERSHIP DEVELOPMENT CHECKLIST

A practical, actionable tool for leaders to track their growth over time and identify areas requiring investment.

C1. Leadership Behaviour Checklist

Tick each statement that reflects your current practice.

Self-Management & Emotional Intelligence

☐ I remain calm under pressure
☐ I recognise my emotional triggers
☐ I reflect on my decisions regularly
☐ I seek feedback from others

Communication

☐ I clearly communicate expectations
☐ I listen actively and without judgement
☐ I adapt communication style to suit the audience
☐ I ensure difficult conversations happen promptly

People Development

☐ I coach and mentor team members
☐ I identify emerging leaders
☐ I delegate effectively
☐ I celebrate staff achievements

Quality & Safety

☐ I use data to guide decisions
☐ I participate in or lead QI initiatives
☐ I promote a just culture
☐ I monitor KPIs routinely

Change & Innovation

☐ I apply structured change methodologies
☐ I actively involve staff in redesign
☐ I evaluate and embed improvements
☐ I remain open to new ideas and technologies

Ethics & Professionalism

☐ I act with fairness and transparency
☐ I maintain professional boundaries
☐ I champion equity and inclusion
☐ I uphold organisational and regulatory standards

C2. Leadership Development Action Plan Template

1. Strengths to Build On

- ____
- ____
- ____

2. Areas for Development

- ____
- ____

3. Actions for the Next 3–6 Months

- Training: _______________________________________
- Mentorship/Coaching: _____________________________
- Stretch Responsibilities: _________________________
- Reflection Focus Areas: ___________________________

4. Evidence of Progress

- KPIs improved?
- Staff feedback?
- 360° feedback themes?
- Achievements or leadership examples?

This action plan can be used in supervision or annual appraisal.

C3. Annual Leadership Capability Review Template

For yearly review or revalidation processes.

Overview

- Role responsibilities
- Significant leadership achievements
- Challenges and how they were managed

Domains

1. Communication

2. Team leadership

3. Operational performance

4. Culture and values

5. Strategic influence

6. Professional conduct

Ratings (1–5)

- 1–2: Needs development
- 3: Competent
- 4: Strong
- 5: Exemplary

Development Priorities for Next Year

- ____
- ____